The Way I See It

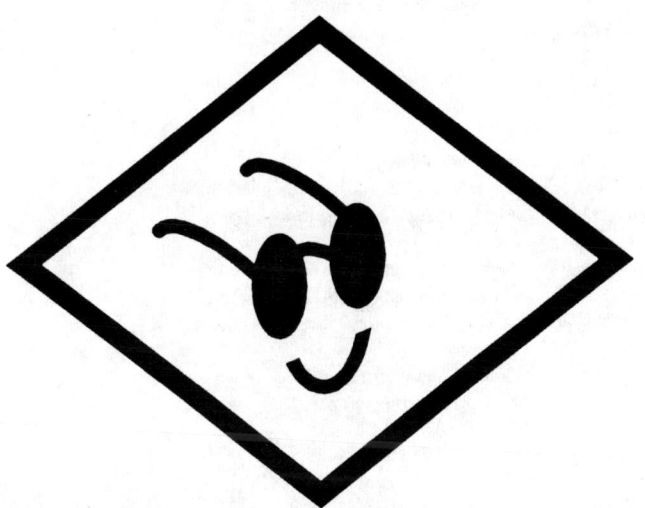

Karen A. Myers, PhD

© Copyright 2004 Karen A. Myers, PhD
All rights reserved. No part of this publication may be reproduced, stored in a retrieval system, or transmitted, in any form or by any means, electronic, mechanical, photocopying, recording, or otherwise, without the written prior permission of the author.

Note for Librarians: a cataloguing record for this book that includes Dewey Decimal Classification and US Library of Congress numbers is available from the Library and Archives of Canada. The complete cataloguing record can be obtained from their online database at:
www.collectionscanada.ca/amicus/index-e.html
ISBN 1-4120-4627-0
Printed in Victoria, BC, Canada

TRAFFORD

Offices in Canada, USA, Ireland, UK and Spain
This book was published *on-demand* in cooperation with Trafford Publishing. On-demand publishing is a unique process and service of making a book available for retail sale to the public taking advantage of on-demand manufacturing and Internet marketing. On-demand publishing includes promotions, retail sales, manufacturing, order fulfilment, accounting and collecting royalties on behalf of the author.

Book sales for North America and international:
Trafford Publishing, 6E–2333 Government St.,
Victoria, BC V8T 4P4 CANADA
phone 250 383 6864 (toll-free 1 888 232 4444)
fax 250 383 6804; email to orders@trafford.com

Book sales in Europe:
Trafford Publishing (UK) Ltd., Enterprise House, Wistaston Road Business Centre, Wistaston Road, Crewe, Cheshire CW2 7RP UNITED KINGDOM
phone 01270 251 396 (local rate 0845 230 9501)
facsimile 01270 254 983; orders.uk@trafford.com

Order online at:
www.trafford.com/robots/04-2435.html

10 9 8 7 6 5 4 3

*Dedicated to
family and friends who are a
part of this book,
especially to
Jim, Kelly, Mom and Dad*

CONTENTS

Introduction 1
Life 5
    Life is Like a Salad Bar 7
Daily Activities 11
    Playing Ball 13
    Knowing Your Colors 15
    Hanging Wallpaper 18
    Watching TV 20
    Making Up 22
    Dancing 25
    Facing People 27
    Voting 29
    Filling Out Forms 31
    The Job Interview 33
Holidays 37
    Easter 39
    Thanksgiving 40
    Christmas 42
Travel 47
    Driving 49
    Flying 51
    Vacation Spots 54
Whispers 61
    Shhh ... She's Blind 63

INTRODUCTION

MINE is a unique family. At least twenty of us are blind. In fact, until I was twenty-four, I was known as the one with the "good" eyes. I could see the street name on the bus, the "Walk/Don't Walk" signs at the crosswalk, the recipe in the cookbook, the phone number on the business card, and the exact color of purple thread to match the purple button on the purple paisley shirt. I even had a driver's license. In the late 1970s all of that changed though, when I, too, was diagnosed with the same hereditary progressive visual disability as everyone else, the one that led to legal blindness.

Fortunately, I grew up around people who considered humor a dietary staple. We continually shared stories about what we could see and what we couldn't see, including the number of parking meters we waved to or bumped into that day, blurting an immediate "excuse me," obviously mistaking them for short, thin pedestrians. We had countless hysterical reenactments of disastrous food buffet escapades where someone mistook mayonnaise for pudding and olive oil for apple juice. I even remember the time when my mother told her three little Catholic children to say "Good morning, Sister" to a nun sitting in a parked car. (This was pre-Vatican Two when nuns still wore elaborate headgear and long veils.) Well, the "nun" turned out to be no nun at all, but rather a tall bucket seat. (The kid with the "good" eyes set Mom straight on that one!)

Living with low vision is definitely a challenge. It also makes life quite adventurous and unpredictable. *The Way I See It* is comprised of 21 tales about me bumping into life. The anecdotes depict some of the adventures I experienced, some of the challenges I faced, and some of the lessons I learned through it all.

For those of you who have ever lost a contact, broken your glasses, experienced your aging parents' Macular Degeneration, or have been in the company of someone who just can't see something, this book may help you remember times when you, too, bumped into life. Each tale ends with a few suggestions to help us get through these situations the next time around.

The way I see it, life is a beautiful gift and we should live it with gusto. Being aware of those around you, respecting their humanity, showing sensitivity to their needs, and sharing laughter and a sense of humor are essentials for life's journey.

LIFE

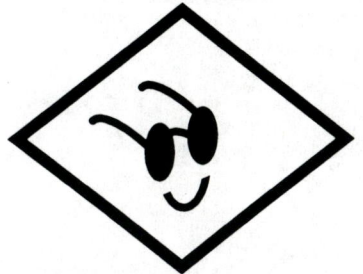

"The Way I See It"

LIFE

Three simple tools for handling life's bumps

LIFE IS LIKE A SALAD BAR

SIMILAR to Forrest Gump's box of chocolates, life with low vision is like going through a salad bar… you never know what you're going to get. At least that's the way I see it. Being legally blind with a progressive visual disability, each day my life becomes a little more like that salad bar.

If you have low vision you can relate to the "joys" of salad bar selection—mistaking pickled beets for spiced apples, black olives for purple grapes, and whipped butter for mustard potato salad. You unknowingly eat hot peppers, parsley, 'hidden' toothpicks, and plastic greenery that was supposed to be decorating the salad bar until it ended up on your plate. And if that wasn't enough, you discover the hard way that the tapioca you took for dessert is horseradish.

As I said, you never know *what* you're going to get. And we're not just talking about salad bars here. The litany of daily concerns continues: Is that the right bus? The right street? The right door? The right restroom? And all this *before* you even get to where you're actually going! Each of us with low vision encounters hundreds of "salad bar shockers" on a daily basis. That's just life with low vision. *Dealing* with life's little surprises is the key.

The way I see it, we (i.e., people with low vision) need three things:

1) **ATTENTIVENESS.** Be aware of your surroundings. Listen.
2) **ASSERTIVENESS.** Ask for assistance. As much as I hate to "bother" people to assist me, I would much rather ask for help than to eat horseradish or end up in the men's restroom—*again*.
3) **A SENSE OF HUMOR.** You gotta laugh! Some of the stuff we do is just too funny. So, take yourself–and your embarrassing moments—lightly.

With the right tools and the right attitude, navigating that salad bar can be as easy as pie (maybe not the whole dessert bar, but definitely the pie).

DAILY ACTIVITIES

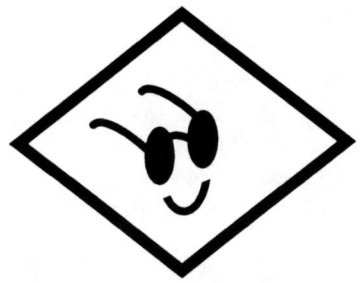

"The Way I See It"

DAILY ACTIVITIES

Managing the day-to-day bumps

PLAYING BALL

"**Let's** play ball!" Oh, dear... there they are. The three most dreaded words in the English language. No, I take that back. There are three even more dreaded words in the English language: "Let's choose teams."

How, you may ask, could any American dread her country's favorite pastime? "Why, it's downright un-American!" they shout from the bleachers (well, okay, maybe from the bleachers in my mind.) But, the truth be known, I *do* dread playing baseball—or any ball for that matter. Why? Because you can only stand being hit in the head so many times.

From little on, no matter what position I played—first base (once), outfield (more than once), or selling popcorn in the stands (by far the safest)—when I heard "Batter up!" my palms began to sweat, my head began to pound, and my heart felt like it was going to leap from my chest. So, what's the big deal? It's called adrenalin, right? Wrong. It's called sheer *terror*! There I was, ducking, covering my head, and praying, "Please don't hit the ball. Please don't hit the ball." Because I didn't want the other team to win? No. Unfortunately, my team spirit wasn't that lofty or loyal. My reason was purely selfish: I didn't want to get hit with the ball—*again*. Nor did I want to hear the moaning and groaning of team members about my clumsiness and obvious "Charlie Brown-like" qualities. You can imagine the panic and fear that overcame many a team captain when they saw me coming their way, which may explain my anti-"Let's choose teams" attitude.

Now, please, don't misunderstand. I know there are people with low vision who love to watch—and play—baseball. And I applaud them. I am a firm believer in achieving your goals, living your dreams, going for the gold, reaching for the stars—and catching them. It's just that high fly ball I have a little trouble with.

KNOWING YOUR COLORS

WHEN did you learn your colors? I can recall sitting in Mrs. Phillip's kindergarten class, attempting to grip an oversized crayon with my tiny fingers while vigorously coloring a picture of a rainbow. ROY-G-BIV. Red, Orange, Yellow, Green, Blue, Indigo, Violet. That's when I learned my colors. I was five. (My daughter, on the other hand, learned her colors at the age of two thanks to Bert and Ernie and the wonders of Sesame Street.) Even though I mastered this task at a relatively young age, isn't it interesting that forty years later I do not seem to know my colors anymore? The fact of the matter is, I do *know* colors; I just am not able to *recognize* them. Low vision has changed a world of vivid colors into grays and tans. But, what's a little less color anyway?

Several years ago, my husband, Jim, and I decided to take advantage of one of the Midwest's sunny fall days by hiking through a state park. As we walked, he kept commenting on the color of the leaves. "Wow, can you see these colors? They're amazing!" he said. "This one's gold, that one's orange, and there's a red one." Obviously, he was in awe. "That's great, Jim," I said in my 'gosh-honey-I'm-so-happy-for-you' voice. I hated to kill the moment by admitting to him that to me those leaves all looked alike, and, if asked to describe them, I would have to say they were all just sort of ...dark. But, don't get me wrong. Even though I couldn't see the leaves' colors, I *could* tell that I was walking through some really big trees and I heard a lot of crunching under my boots—which I assumed were dried leaves. I'd hate to think they were a swarm of locusts or a herd of roaches or gaggle of really big ants. My point is that I had a lot of fun hiking that day, leaves or no leaves.

While discussing our weekend adventures around the proverbial water cooler (i.e., in the women's john), a very puzzled co-worker asked me a rather legitimate question: "How can you enjoy walking in the woods if you can't see anything?" "Well," I replied, "I guess I enjoy it in the same way I enjoy a parade, a circus, or a ballet—through all my senses, even sight (limited as it may be). I enjoy just being there."

After overhearing our conversation, my new administrative assistant, Debbie, later approached me. "I didn't realize you were colorblind," she said, almost apologetically. "I thought you *wanted* to sign all those letters in **RED** ink." As my face became the color of the pen I mistakenly used, she quickly added, "Why don't I put a piece of tape around your red pens so you can feel the difference?" Yes! Great idea! Easy, efficient, effective, and inexpensive. Now that's my kind of assistant! Hey, maybe she could "code" my sock drawer—or, better yet, my entire closet. Do you think that would be stretching that phrase in her job description, "Other duties as assigned?" I suppose there is only one way to find out..."Oh, Debbie, could you come here, please?"

HANGING WALLPAPER

HAVE you ever caught yourself staring at the wall deep in thought, contemplating the secrets of the universe, when all of a sudden you hear yourself asking, "Who in the world hung this wallpaper? It's a mess!"— which brings me to yet another escapade, "The Adventures of the Three Blind Wallpaper Hangers."

Once upon a time, there was a woman with extremely low vision who wanted to sell her house so she could move to a new city in another state far far away. To "spruce up" her house before putting it on the market, the woman asked her younger sister (with even lower vision) and her mother (with even lower lower vision) to help her. In the midst of cleaning and fixing and in a moment of creative lunacy, the youngest of the trio suggested they wallpaper the bathroom (probably because they destroyed the walls while ripping off the old wallpaper, making painting a non-option). The women selected a textured white paper, virtually impossible to screw up—or so they "blindly" believed. Unfortunately, the paper did have a slight pattern undetected by the women, and the three blind wallpaper hangers made a few minor errors. When the sighted husbands of the three blind wallpaper hangers were summoned to enter the room and admire their wives' handiwork, a horrified gasp filled the air. For after 12 hours of highly intense labor accompanied by hysterical laughter, the three blind wallpaper hangers hung a totally mismatched bathroom. Well, at least we (er, I mean *they*) had a good time, right?

The moral of the story is this: 1) Don't quit your day job, ladies. 2) Beware of wallpaper hangers with low vision (at least the three I know). 3) In case you're in the market for a house in Georgia, I can get you a great deal on one with a slightly imperfect white bathroom. Now, won't you please sing along (to the tune of *Three Blind Mice*)...

Three blind wallpaper hangers.
Three blind wallpaper hangers.
See how they paste. See how they paste.
They dip and they hang and they brush and they wipe,
Patterns and textures and solids and stripe,
Nothing matches but what's the big gripe?
They're three blind wallpaper hangers.

WATCHING TV

"**Hey,** Mom, move your head! You're blocking the screen!" Now, there's a sweet request, one I've heard almost daily ever since my darling daughter, Kelly, learned to watch TV and utter commands at the same time. A familiar sight in my house is me, an avid movie buff with extremely low vision, sitting six inches from the TV set squinting desperately at the picture. But, hey, as long as I am close enough to the screen and the lighting is just right, I'm in TV heaven. Luckily, my understanding family has learned to patiently crane their necks and watch around me (except for that one night when I heard them furiously emptying Kelly's piggy bank and muttering something about buying a second TV or two neck braces).

My mom (the wonderful woman who generously passed her low vision and positive outlook onto me and my siblings), on the other hand, discovered an excellent alternative to squinting at the screen: audio descriptive videos. With audio description, a voice describes the action as the movie progresses. For example, as the camera moves in on the scarecrow in the field, the voice says, "Dorothy sees a scarecrow in a cornfield." The voice-over is inserted into the existing audio intending not to override the dialog.

The great thing is that Mom can borrow descriptive videos through the public library, so she can "watch" her favorite movies for *free* from across the room without sitting on top of the set (unlike some people we know). I realize I should follow my mother's example and look into audio descriptive videos. But, that incessant optimism inherited from my maternal grandmother tells me that if I hold out a little longer, that accommodating family of mine will get tired of craning their necks, let loose of those pennies, and surprise me with a 72-inch plasma screen. In the meantime, my big head shall remain in their sight line.

MAKING UP

"**Aw,** screw this makeup! I'd rather not wear any makeup at all than to have my face look like it was done by my two-year old with finger paints!" Sound familiar? I've known many women with low vision who gave up on makeup because it's just too difficult to apply. After all, who needs that hassle? Well, let me tell you a little story that just might change your mind. [Gentlemen, I realize that this topic may be the least of your worries. But, if you want to make some brownie points, share this with your female friends, because, believe me, women DO know what I'm talking about.]

I always dreamed of becoming an actress. I performed wherever they let me—from living rooms and church basements to huge auditoriums and amphitheatres. Raw talent unleashed itself in a variety of roles ranging from Gypsy Rose Lee, the renowned "exotic" dancer (a light stretch for me) to Snoopy, Charlie Brown's sophisticated canine (obviously type-casting).

Part of the fun of amateur theatre is doing your own makeup. And one of the neat things about stage makeup is that even if you can't see too well, it's fairly easy to apply and difficult to mess up—or, if you do, it's hardly noticeable (except to the people in the first row).

Applying makeup in real life, however, is a whole other story. With less than 20/20 vision (or, in my case, 20/200), the "squint and pray" method of makeup application is how it gets done. Barely seeing my own reflection in the mirror, I would apply blotchy foundation and clumpy mascara all for the sake of beauty. Beauty? Yeah, right. More like *Zombie Bride: The Sequel.* Over the years, I spent hundreds—probably thousands—of dollars searching for the "right" products. Then one sleepless night a few years ago I found the answer on, of all places, an infomercial. Yes, folks, that's right. In the wee hours of the morning, I discovered sheer, pre-matched worry-free makeup complete with "how-to" video. For the first time in my life, my makeup matched and I was actually complimented in broad daylight on my makeup artistry. Now that is something to sing about.

The way I see it, we do not need to turn in our cosmetic case key just because we have low vision. We just need to know the process. In my case, I started out with the infomercial product, the video, and a high powered magnified mirror. I then progressed to the skincare salon, which I found extremely beneficial. The key is to explain your visual limitations to the makeup or skincare specialist, discuss your options, and experiment in the store and at home. If the products don't work and you don't feel comfortable with their performance, return them and try again. I never thought makeup would be possible with my visual acuity, but I stand corrected.

As the man says, "All the world's a stage." Now I can do my own makeup, play my daily role, and not worry about the people in the front row seats. How's that for perfection? I do believe my dream has come true.

DANCING

I love to dance and always have. In fact, with thirteen years of training, I once considered going professional with the dance thing. As I got older, though, dance lessons became difficult for me. I began feeling awkward and embarrassed in front of my classmates. I stayed away from dance classes, and, on the rare occasion I did attempt group lessons, I looked and felt as though I had the grace of Bigfoot. So, what happened to me? Where did all that talent go?

Just about the time I decided my dance learning curve had taken its final dip, it hit me. "I've got it!" I screamed (which was rather embarrassing since I was in the supermarket line at the time). The reason was so simple. Because I couldn't see the teacher, I wasn't learning the correct steps. And because I didn't know the correct steps, I appeared unpolished, ungraceful, and downright uncoordinated. The problem wasn't in my ability to dance but rather in the instructional process itself. The solution? One-on-one dance lessons.

Yes, it's true. I recently learned to swing dance in a small group with the instructor right in front of me and often dancing with me. So, dancers of the world, move aside because the Queen of Swing is back on the floor!

Not long ago, I witnessed an amazing performance by the Cleveland Ballet Dancing Wheels, a dance company of standing and sitting dancers (dancers who use wheelchairs). As part of their show, three people with disabilities from our own community performed with them, including a friend of mine who is totally blind. My friend, who did a lovely job despite his innate clumsiness, told us that the key to his successful debut was the creativity of the choreographer and his sighted partner. Both teachers were creative in their training techniques, and they taught him in such a way that he could learn the movements without actually seeing the instructor. The result was phenomenal.

The way I see it, creative thinking is what accommodating people with visual disabilities is all about. From talking signs to one-on-one dance lessons, doing things a little differently, thinking out of the box, is all it takes to give us the opportunity, the confidence, and the choice to sit it out or dance. I choose to *dance*!

FACING PEOPLE

"*How embarrassing! I'll never be able to show my face in public again.*" Sound familiar? All of us at some time or another (some of us at more times than we wish to admit) have done something embarrassing. In particular, those of us with low vision have an uncanny knack for social blunders largely because we can't see what we look like.

For example, there was the time in high school when I wore two different shoes to school. After I discovered my fashion faux pas during third period Latin class (for some reason I was staring at my feet rather than the conjugations on the blackboard), I spent the rest of the day hysterically explaining to my peers (most of whom could care less) how hastily I dressed that morning.

Speaking of embarrassing moments, a friend told me that she noticed a man who was blind walking down the street with a very long trail of tissue stuck to his shoe. She didn't know what to say, so she tried to sneak up behind him and stomp the tissue with her own foot. But every time she attempted to stomp it, the man walked faster. She said the man seemed startled. (Imagine that. He probably couldn't figure out why some woman was stomping bugs so closely behind him.) A perfect example of why the sneak approach is rarely successful.

And, just the other day, a colleague discovered a 37-cent postage stamp in my hair. It apparently had attached itself to the earpiece of my sunglasses while in my purse—a sticky situation to say the least.

So, what is a person to do? The way I see it, if you have low vision you must *ask* people how you look, if you are presentable, if your colors match, etc, etc, etc. If you see a person with low vision in one of these embarrassing predicaments, politely and quietly inform him or her of the problem. Nine times out of ten (and most often, ten times out of ten), the person will be ever so thankful for your kindness, sensitivity and honesty. Remember, no matter how embarrassing the situation, you can always show your face again, but you'll feel a lot better if you're one hundred percent sure that when you do, you don't have blueberries in your teeth and post-it notes on your chin.

VOTING

TODAY is Election Day. Today is the culmination of months (which seem like years) of active campaigning, fundraising, and vote gathering. Today is the day we exercise our constitutional right, let our voices be heard, rock the vote, and make our vote count. Today is the day I walk into a very bright room and go behind a tiny little curtain to punch a tiny little hole next to a tiny little name on a tiny little card. Today is the day I panic.

What if I rock the vote the wrong way? It's not that I'm undecided. I know for which candidates I plan to vote. But, as a person with low vision, I am always concerned whether or not my stylus hits the appropriate mark or my finger hits the intended key. Does anyone else ever worry about this?

Now you may say, "Why don't you ask someone for help? After all, according to the law, accommodations must be made to ensure equal access." This is true; however, there is this very private, and, I must sadly admit, very vain part of me that insists on doing it myself. Does anyone else feel this way?

Today is also the day that all the campaign signs come down—you know, all those election promos that scream,

Vote for Groat, I like Pike, Stan's your Man, and *All the way with Jay.* Some people see them as cluttering up the scenery. I, on the other hand, use them as visual markers—political bread crumbs, if you will—to find my way home. I turn right at *Stan's your Man,* left at *I like Pike,* and when I see *Jay,* I know I'm almost all the way to my front door. Oh, how I will miss those catchy slogans plastered all over lawns and billboards. I can only hope that these lovely lawn indicators will be rapidly replaced with "House for Sale" or "Insulation Inside" signs to prevent me from getting lost in the woods, or, at best, walking into someone else's living room.

But, back to the voting booth. My biggest concern today is punching the wrong dot on the ballot. The names look so similar to me, how can I tell the difference? Should I ask for help or will my vanity cost us the election? "Mirror, Mirror, on the wall, who's the fairest candidate of them… Oh my gosh, you're right, I *do* need a facial! Now where's that spa number?"

FILLING OUT FORMS

"**S**IGN this permission slip." "Read and edit attached report." "Sign and return enclosed insurance forms."

These are typical daily messages. No big deal, right?—unless, of course, you can't see them. When you have low vision, like I do, each written message automatically presents challenges:

1. Is the message readable? Or is it scribbled in pencil on paper the size of a postage stamp?
2. Is the task itself readable? That is, once I decipher the message, am I able to see the number in the phone book, the photocopied permission slip, the report draft, and the insurance form? Probably not.

After years of squinting and pretending I could see hand-written messages—and ultimately missing a few too many appointments and deadlines—I came up with several ways to ensure *readability*.

- ✓ I give a felt-tip pen to anyone who writes me notes on a regular basis.
- ✓ When people write me notes "on the spot," I ask them to use my felt-tip marker and "print BIG."

- ✓ I request all documents, reports and bills in large print.
- ✓ I use a hand-held magnification reader as well as one that connects to my television or computer monitor and magnifies reading material, photos, and even sewing needles.

The way I see it, we need to educate ourselves and others about low vision "tricks of the trade" to make life a little easier on the eyes.

THE JOB INTERVIEW

IT is 8:45 a.m. I hit the "UP" button and nervously await the elevator that will take me to the fourth floor. On the ride up, the mental debate continues. My interview is less than thirteen minutes away and I still haven't made a decision: Should I or should I not tell them that I have low vision? If I do tell them, it may hurt my chances for getting the job. Although I know quite well that legally they can't discriminate based on disability, I can't seem to suppress that nagging fear that if I tell them, I'll blow it. On the other hand, if I don't tell them about my vision, I will be hiding the "real" me. Although my vision is neither my identity nor my character, it is indeed a large part of who I am and how I communicate. Nine minutes to go. What should I do?

The scenario you just read is true. In fact, it happened to me twice within a two-month period. So, what was my decision? Did I choose to disclose or not to disclose my disability? The answer is: Both. In my first interview, I did not disclose. I decided to discuss my qualifications and vision for the job, but not mention my own vision (or lack thereof). I donned my dark glasses from time to time to read my notes, but never mentioned why I was wearing them. Unable to see my interviewers' faces, I couldn't read or respond to their nonverbals, a behavior that may have negatively affected our interaction. At the end of the eight-hour interview process, I left feeling uncomfortable about my choice not to disclose. I did not get the job.

In the next interview one month later, I did disclose my visual disability, and I can't tell you how comfortable and relieved I felt. I let them see "me" (even though I couldn't see them!), and I was able to use humor about my vision to put them at ease. Did I get the job? Unfortunately, no. The experience, however, left me with the confidence and conviction to "tell it like it is" during my next interview, and yes, I did get the job!

Note: Just so we're clear about this, to me "telling it like it is" means telling them about my low vision. When it comes to age (although illegal to ask), that's a horse of a different color. I'm 39 and sticking to it. I do have my standards.

HOLIDAYS

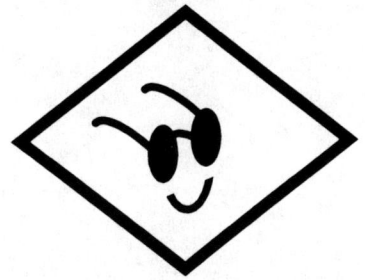

"The Way I See It"

HOLIDAYS

Bumping into special occasions

EASTER

THANKS to Punxsutawney Phil who did *not* see his shadow on February 2, Groundhog Day, Spring is on its way.

Spring is my favorite season—a time of hope, cleansing, and rebirth; days chock full of sounds and smells (important elements to those of us with low vision)—like chirping robins, fragrant daffodils, and fresh-cut grass. Spring also brings Easter, which of course means indulging in the infamous Easter Egg Hunt.

Now, the great Easter Egg Hunt in my family is indeed a sight to behold. There's nothing more amusing than a slew of squinting egg hunters decked out in big dark glasses sniffing out the colorful treats that are conveniently camouflaged by the thick dewy lawn. Is that an egg? I pick it up, sniff it, and discover it is only a rock. What about this one? Crunch. Yep, that *was* one, but now I know what they mean when they say "walking on eggshells." At least they are not crazy enough to use cream-filled ones. Squish. Hmmm, I'm afraid I spoke too soon. Remind me next year not to wear sandals.

THANKSGIVING

"**Let's** talk turkey." Now, there's an old expression for you. It usually means, "Let's get down to business," "Let's cut to the chase" or, in more contemporary circles, "Let's get to the bottom line." In my house on a Thanksgiving Day not too long ago, however, it meant something entirely different.

It all began on a cool crisp November morning. The family was coming to our house around two o'clock for Thanksgiving dinner. The turkey had spent the night in a bucket of cold water in the garage. No, not my husband… the *other* turkey. I spent the morning preparing all the trimmings—you know, the essentials like Stove Top Stuffing (turkey flavor), Heinz Homestyle Gravy (turkey flavor), Ore-Ida real mashed potatoes (once frozen but still very real), Ocean Spray Cranberry Sauce (maintaining that can-like shape on the plate which is amazing in itself), and homemade bread (sure it is—as long as I hide the bag). Oh, and I can't forget my friend Sara Lee who so graciously provided her perfect pumpkin pie. As you can tell, I worked long and hard on my scrumptious feast, selecting just the right box, can, jar, and bag to complement the star of the show, Mr. Butterball himself, Tom T. Turkey. Now, the great thing about turkey cooking is those cool plastic cooking bags. You put a little flour in the bag (yes, I know what flour is, I just don't use it for anything else like *baking*), add a little water, throw in the turkey, stick it in a pan, and voila! In a few hours you have a beautiful scrumptious golden brown entree. And that's just what I did. At precisely 11 a.m., I assisted Tom into the oven chamber. He proceeded to cook for 2 hours and 45 min. At 1:45 p.m., my husband placed Tom on the serving platter and began slicing—or rather, he attempted the slicing process. I'm afraid Tom was a tad tough. Half-frozen is probably more accurate. What could have gone wrong? I followed all the directions: flour, water, bird in bag, slits, oven—ah, the oven. The oven and those tricky little dials. You know, it's amazing how similar the words "Bake" and "Broil" look to the human eye, isn't it? After all, they both do begin with "B." All right! I admit it! I did it! I BROILED the turkey! Lucky for me, most of the people in my family can't see too well, so they weren't too disgusted by Tom's pink pallor.

My oh-so-loving family refuses to let me forget that day—the day I discovered how helpful a tactile indicator (a raised dot, perhaps) on the word "Bake" might be, and the day that the phrase, "Let's talk turkey" became a reality since *talking* was about all we could do with it. Eating definitely was out of the question.

CHRISTMAS

IF you're dreaming of a white Christmas, you might not want to come to our house for the holidays. If you did, you would find the traditional Currier and Ives snow and sledding replaced with sun and surfing Beach Boys style.

Although we've lived on the east coast, in the Midwest, and in the southwest, we quickly discovered that west coast living, particularly life in southern California, is quite different. For one thing, clouds are a rarity and sunshine is the norm, which means curtainless windows, wide-open doors, and year-round outdoor activities. For someone who is extremely light sensitive, this new sunny lifestyle was a challenge for me. Sunglasses became a regular—and necessary—part of my daily wardrobe. Lucky for me, the "shades" look works in So Cal.

As a child in Illinois, I would peek out the window on Christmas morning, thrilled to discover the six inches of snow that had fallen during the night. Now, as an adult in California, I throw open the patio door on Christmas morning and step out into 75 degree weather. And keeping with a new family tradition, I shout, "Grab the sunscreen, we're off to the beach!"

One of my favorite memories is walking barefoot in the sand with my beaming 79-year old mother, collecting seashells and chasing waves, while my beaming 84-year-old dad waved to us proudly from his beach chair. (Well, at least I *think* that was my dad waving. I guess it could have been a very large seagull flapping its wings or a big umbrella swaying back and forth in the sand or...) Anyway, this was their first time to the Pacific Ocean and their enthusiasm was contagious. I, too, was beaming and thrilled to be their seaside guide.

Mom and I share the same eyes, that is, we both have hazel eyes that are legally blind. And even though we couldn't see the sailboat on the horizon or the color of the surfer's suit (okay, I admit we couldn't even see the surfer), we *could* see and experience that magnificent ocean. Feeling the warmth of the sun on our faces, smelling the salty air, hearing the excitement in my mother's voice as she discovered yet another shell... just sharing these moments with my family was worth all the squinting and all the missed snowflakes in the world.

The way I see it, home is where the heart is and happiness is where you find it. And no matter what color Christmas is or what coast or continent you happen to be on, sharing the holiday spirit with people you love, whether you see them or not, is what it's all about.

TRAVEL

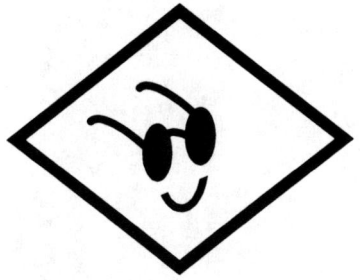

"The Way I See It"

TRAVEL

Bumping into roads, clouds, and hot spots

DRIVING

My vision was pretty decent at 16. So decent, in fact, that I received my driver's license that year. (Well, okay, maybe not on the first try. I did speed through that school zone at 22 mph, which had nothing to do with my vision but rather, as my father informed me, something to do with the weight of my foot.) My point is that I could see quite well at 16. Eight short years later, however, I voluntarily gave up the privilege of driving for my own safety and the safety of all other drivers and pedestrians. When I no longer could distinguish between red, yellow, and green traffic lights or see workmen holding signs expecting— then begging—me to STOP, I knew it was time to throw in the keys. Although it's difficult to relinquish the wheel, life does go on, and as I quickly discovered, I must go on with it. I could not allow the inability to drive to hinder my life's goals and ambitions.

As a result, at the age of 24 I found a whole new set of friends who helped me live life to the fullest. And no matter where I lived from that time on (ten different cities to date, from east coast to west coast), those friends travel with me. Although their names and faces may change with each city, their importance to me is unwavering. So, who are these crucial companions, the ones who make my day-to-day travel possible? They are my punctual pals, my constant comrades—the bus driver, the taxi driver, the subway operator, and those dear friends with cars.

The way I see it, if you are unable to drive in this world of taken for-granted license-holders, then you must use your imagination and your resources to get where you need to go. If you can't see the number on the bus, the door on the taxi, or even your friend's big red SUV (which apparently is the size of a garbage truck), let those new-found travel guides know that you need their help. This help may range from informing you of the bus number or its destination, to meeting you at your door, to escorting you to the vehicle, or, in the case of the friend in the big red SUV, yelling, "Hey, Karen, it's me, Ruth. Get in!" Believe me, once these folks know you are an independent person who is asking them—actually counting on them—to assist you to your destination, most will be happy to oblige. (Throwing in a little gas money or offering to pay for lunch from time to time doesn't hurt either!)

Although this part of your venture does take initiative and self-advocacy, it is well worth it. By using your own creativity and resources, and by asking for and accepting the assistance of your license-bearing friends, you, too, may proudly announce, "Keys or no keys, I have arrived!"

FLYING

MORE often than not, I fly solo; that is, I fly without a sighted companion. For a person with low vision, traveling alone is a challenge, and for me, it's a real anxiety-booster. I don't have a fear of flying, mind you; I just have a fear of going to the wrong gate, missing signs, and getting on the wrong plane.

People in the airline industry relate to people with visual disabilities in various ways. The reservation agent on the phone is usually very friendly and accommodating (after all, the final sale is pending at that stage of the game). Upon describing my need for flight assistance due to my visual disability, the reservation agent promptly enters my request into the computer and assures me that my needs will be met. Arriving at the airport, however, is another story.

If the luck of the Irish is with me that day, my shuttle driver escorts me to the appropriate terminal door which means that, more often than not, I ask anyone passing by to point me in the direction of my airline entrance. Once in the airport, locating my airline counter or rather my airline "line" (i.e., queue) is a major ordeal. I ask friendly fliers or airport personnel where to go.

As I stand in line waiting for my turn at the ticket counter (or worse, the self-serve computer), one thought keeps rushing through my mind: When one of the ticket agents yells "Next!" how will I know when that "next" is me? This particular step in the flying process is extremely nerve-wracking.

With luggage checked and boarding pass in hand, I make my way to "the gates." This entails finding the security checkpoint labeled "Open" (because going through a closed one is not only pointless but extremely embarrassing). It also involves maneuvering my belongings (e.g., purse, carry-on, camera, white cane, coat, shoes, etc.) on to the conveyor belt, and then quickly retrieving my belongings before being bombarded by bundles behind me. Squinting and searching for my gate is next. And once I find the gate itself, locating the gate check-in counter, the appropriate waiting area, and finally, the actual door to the airplane confirms that the fun never stops. Usually at this point in my journey, a restroom is welcome; however, finding the right entrance (you know, Men, Women, Maintenance Closet) may require precious moments not included in my travel schedule.

I often pre-board with children, people with special needs, and those in first-class. Flight attendants tend to be extremely friendly at this stage of the trek. In fact, some tend to go overboard to ensure my comfort. There are those who speak loudly to compensate for my vision loss (because we all know that people who are blind are also deaf, right?). There are those who speak slowly to me to compensate for my loss of mental capacity (because we all know that people with low vision have low IQs, no?). And there are those who speak in a child-like manner to compensate for who-knows-what (but, just as long as they bring me a pair of those little plastic wings, who cares!). Some flight attendants go through the safety instructions with me one-on-one; some describe the food on my plate in great detail; some make sure my glass is always full; and others insist on fluffing my pillow. It never fails, though. After catering to my every (sightless) need, each one of them presents me with an armful of the latest publications, and, while moving my white cane aside, asks sweetly, "Would you like something to read?"

The way I see it, for stress-free solo flying, ask the airline for personal assistance from the time you reach the airport for departure until the time you leave the airport upon arrival. This sure-fire stress reliever is as good as a scented candle and a hot bath.

VACATION SPOTS

Question: What do seven pairs of glasses, a purse big enough to hold seven pairs of glasses, and *Dramamine* have in common?
Answer: Me on a trip.

Trip #1: Colorado

Not long ago I attended a five-day leadership institute in Colorado. As a person with low vision, traveling alone or with colleagues can be quite an adventure, and, believe me, this was. It all began with me achieving one of my greatest feats: finding a purse large enough to hold my collection of glasses yet light enough to carry on my 18-hour day treks. Since I have to use specific lenses for specific tasks depending on the lighting—and since no one has yet invented an all-in-one pair of glasses for me (big hint to inventors out there)—I carry at least seven pairs of glasses with me at all times. Luckily, I found the perfect bag in the nick of time.

Despite having the perfect bag and 50 hilarious companions, challenges did raise their prickly little heads. As I reflect on those five fun-filled days, I thought it was only fair to share with you some traveler's words of wisdom—or should I say traveler's words of *warning*...

Advice for Travelers in Colorado (or anywhere else for that matter)
1. Beware of crossing a busy street with "friends" who forget to tell you when they are going to *dash* across. Standing alone in the middle of a busy intersection can be a tad disturbing.
2. Beware of clear plastic cups filled with clear beverages displayed on a sun-drenched white tablecloth. These cups become invisible and are easy targets when you're reaching for the cocktail weenies.
3. Beware of mountains. Although they may be pretty to people who can see them, hiking alone in search of inner peace may be hazardous to your health (and to the health of any small creature in your path).
4. Beware of elk, deer, horses, and mountain goats. They all look alike, including the droppings they leave behind.
5. Beware of the hygiene paper strip over the toilet seat. It'll get ya every time.

Trip #2: Las Vegas

As most first-time tourists in Vegas, I was overwhelmed not only by the bright lights, glitz and glamour of the city that never sleeps, but also by the millions of people on the streets 24 hours a day, which makes it a bit challenging for someone who can't see too well. Talk about stimuli overload. Whether I was on the Strip, at a casino, in a buffet line, in the bright sunlight, or amid the pulsating Vegas lights, I continually bumped into bodies, stepped on toes, dashed in front of cars, and crashed into baby strollers. I soon discovered that walking and sightseeing definitely were not my forte in this city.

So, I thought I'd play it safe and stay close to my newfound friends, the slot machines. But even they tricked me with their multitude of buttons, bells, whistles, and flashing lights not to mention that some of them wanted nickels, others required quarters, and still others demanded half-dollars. What a nightmare. I kept putting the wrong coins in the wrong slots and then wondered why I never won. (Yes, a few lucky souls actually *do* win in Vegas. Not me, mind you, but a few lucky souls.)

The way I see it, when you are visiting Las Vegas and you have low vision, you need to do two things: 1) take a sighted travel companion with you. I must admit that I trampled far fewer people when Jim was with me. He's great at "steering" me away from the masses; and 2) ask Luck to be a lady not only at night but in the morning and afternoon as well. Luck definitely comes in handy when you are trying to find your hotel room and distinguish between a 50-cent and a $5.00 slot machine. It's amazing how similar those two numbers look in lights. And, by the way, if you're wondering just how well I did at the casinos, let's just say that the one-arm bandits lived up to their reputations.

Trip #3: The San Diego Zoo

Eureka! I found it! Finally, something I can see ... the *elephant* at the San Diego Zoo! And, if the lighting is just right, I can see the giraffe, the rhino, the hippo, the gorilla, the giant panda, and the polar bear. Yes, I realize that these are the largest animals in the zoo. And, yes, I also realize that I can't even begin to locate or recognize the other 4,000 zoo inhabitants (from aardvarks to zebras). But to be able to see these huge animals up close and personal in what appears to be their natural habitat—well, that's just cool.

Trip #4: Mackinac Island (my favorite place)

Mackinac Island, in Michigan's Upper Peninsula, is my favorite place in the world. It is the perfect stress-free zone for people with low vision because all motor vehicles (low vision nightmares) are prohibited. Yes, prohibited. Automobiles are replaced by horse-drawn carriages and bicycles. It's as if you stepped back in time, and to me, it is the ideal environment.

Jim and I like to ride a bicycle-built-for-two around the

island, a common mode of transportation. Tandem bikes are perfect for me because I get to enjoy the scenery and breeze on the back while Jim does all the navigating—and pedaling—from the front. Another favorite pastime is eating island fudge followed by another ride around the island to work off all those decadent calories.

Although Mackinac (pronounced Mack-uh-naw) Island is, well, *perfect*, there are two things I feel I should warn you about. One is Suzy, the mare with the attitude. Jim and I took her—er, rather, she took us–on a white-knuckled buggy ride that scared the living daylights out of me. Obviously, she knew what she was doing and didn't want any part of Jim's "reigning." My advice is to steer clear of Suzy.

The other warning is to watch out for what Suzy and her comrades leave behind. I suppose that's the downside of horses—watching where you step. My advice is to take a sighted companion to share the tranquility and help you avoid the Suzy "surprises." With a little gracious guidance, you can bravely step back in time without boldly stepping in "it."

WHISPERS

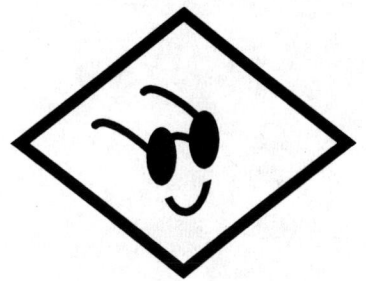

"The Way I See It"

WHISPERS

Things that go bump in the light

SHHH...SHE'S BLIND

WHY is it that people "clam up" when they are around a person with a visible visual disability (i.e. those of us with low or no vision who wear dark lenses, use assistive aids and devices, carry white canes, or are accompanied by guide dogs)? Case in point: One sunny day I was walking through the atrium of a public building, sporting my dark glasses and white cane. (My cane comes in handy in a particularly bright environment.) As I approached a group of people engaged in light and lively conversation, an abrupt hush fell over the crowd. Not a sound. You actually could hear the proverbial pin drop. What happened? Where did they go? I was doing just fine up until then. Their voices were guiding me and I was "listening" to where they were standing so I wouldn't plow into them. Then all of a sudden—silence. It was as if they disappeared. They not only stopped talking, they stopped breathing! I strained to hear a wheeze, a cough, a snort—but nothing. Finally, I heard a faint whisper, "Jack, get out of the way." It occurred to me that I was about to smack Jack with my cane. I wonder if he would have let out a yelp if I did. I made it past the mum group (or maybe it was the mime troupe), thinking to myself how nice it would have been if they had continued talking to each other as I approached or if one of them said "Hello!" to me. Either way I would have known someone was there and gauged my path of travel accordingly.

These "hush" episodes (as I so fondly call them) occur on a daily basis. I recall relaying one of these episodes to Kelly when she was sixteen. It happened at work that day and involved five "whispering" professors who apparently thought I had "low hearing" as well as low vision. My daughter just shook her head in disbelief. Later that evening she gave me this poem. Insightful, no?

"Shhh... She's BLIND"
She walks into the room tapping her cane.
All mouths immediately close.
In a room full of people she is alone
and no one thinks she knows.

People feel pity for this woman,
which seems so absurd to me.
For even though the eyes are blind
cannot the mind still see?

She has the ability to think and speak.
Oh yes, all this she can do.
And go ahead—try to tiptoe around her

but don't think she cannot hear you.

This is a 37-year-old woman.
Stop treating her like she's four.
She can walk and think on her own,
and she's capable of opening her own door.

You know this woman is independent.
You know she has an intelligent mind.
Yet when she enters that "empty" room
you still turn to whisper, "Shhh... She's BLIND."

Kelly L. Myers, Age 16

ISBN 1-41204627-0